I have Crabs, Gas and some other Shit!

by

Larry A. Yff

My last couple of books read like a conversation and I'm liking that style more and more. When I have Chapters, an Introduction, a Summary and a Table of Contents I get claustrophobic. I feel inhibited...I think.

I feel inhibited if that means "stuck". I like to ramble a bit and Conversation Style writing allows me to do that. Did you see how I capitalized it and tried to make that style look official? Like it's really a thing?

Anyways, I was thinking about all the natural resources we have on the planet and how far in advance they were put here and that's where the ideal for this book sprang up. Somebody placed everything we need on this planet waaaay before us humans got here, but, in our everyday grind to consume and use these resources to make as much money as we can...most of us don't have time to think about such things.

Lucky for you, I have that kind of time right now as a starving author. I have time to stare out the window, think about some shit, listen to the Holy Spirit put some better shit into my head and then write what He tells me to write.

I guess that's more or less my Introduction, so we might as well get the rest of the conversation started. I think this is what you would officially call The Body of this book...

Crabs. I told you I have crabs and I do. Well, I have access to crabs, shrimp, oysters and lobster and yes, I also *had* crabs, but we'll start with the food crab and work our way to the sexually-transmitted-disease crab.

What does this have to do with this topic of acknowledging God in creation? A whole lot. Let me show you...

I had a friend of mine recently tell me He believed in God, but He didn't feel the need to follow His laws since there are so many of them and the majority of them don't make any sense.

Since he is in to homosexual activity, he obviously included this on his list of "no sense" laws from God.

He gave a couple of examples he thought were extreme and one had to do with shrimp. He said God told us not to eat seafoods like shrimp, but we do anyways. I had to agree with him, but we didn't get into a big argument 'cause that's not my thing. I can agree to disagree.

Netta is into culinary stuff and she once told me shrimp, one of my favorite foods, was a bottom-feeder. She said they eat shit off the bottom of the sea and it's because of that, they actually are dirty animals that shouldn't be eaten...we agreed to disagree.

We disagreed until I did some "First 48" detective work and it led me, once again, to the realization that somebody was again trying to get my attention away from God and His laws for some reason. I put on my detective hat and badge and began to find out who would do this and why...

Stop and think about the most expensive foods on any menu. What types of foods come to mind? I'll bet seafood comes to mind.

Typically, you are going to pay top dollar for shrimp, lobster or crab dishes. Since they are so expensive, it makes people want to buy them more. Why? Is it because they have an irresistible taste?

I agree these foods taste good, but at the same time, I have to acknowledge they are shitty foods to eat and probably aren't the best for our bodies. I mean, seriously, any animals that literally eat shit off the ocean floor or decaying fish probably aren't the best for us. What do you think?

What do you think and why is that important? It's important because of their price and diet. People are going crazy trying to catch and kill as many lobsters, crabs and shrimp as possible to make as much money as possible.

What's happening is without millions of these bottom-feeders, the sea is collecting tons of shit and rotting fish. It's as though every form of life on the planet is designed to carry out a certain function as part of a plan. Hmmm, doesn't that kind of lead to a designer or a creator or planner of Earth?

Making those seafood animals expensive also drives up the need for people to buy them. I don't think it's so much the taste as it is the "rich appeal". People who can afford these types of food feel rich. They feel superior. They feel like they have exquisite and expensive taste when in reality, they are eating the shit-eating janitors of the sea!

This seems like a common theme when dealing with Satan: he takes the stuff that is bad for us and makes it look appealing and desirable. I seriously never looked at it from that view and I guess I was content to not make that discovery because yes, shrimp and lobster *was* very appealing, desirable and tasty!

When I began to look at seafood and God's laws from a different view, I began to think: maybe God was looking out for our health? Maybe He was acknowledging the fact these animals existed, but that He designed some animals to be eaten and some to perform other tasks.

Let's take a moment to look at the other crabs. The ones that are the result of sexually-transmitted diseases…and yes, I had those too!

I love talking about sex and sex-related topics because the understanding of sex and our bodies is the number one step towards understanding the purpose of humanity.

I used to believe all sin was the same, but then I came across several manuscripts that said sexual sins were the exception. Sexual sins use the body to sin; while the other sins like murder use objects like guns and knives.

I know, I said I have crabs and I'm about to get there. Give me a little time...

So, one of the authors of the Bible records God as saying the body is not designed for sexual immorality. In other words, when you use the body for sex in the wrong way, bad shit can physically happen...like you might get crabs in your crotch like I did! Check this out...

This is something about sex that didn't make sense to me until I discovered what I just told you about God saying the body isn't meant for sex outside His rules for sex.

I didn't understand how I could have no sexually transmitted disease (STD) and let's say my friend Jane didn't have any either. Her and I have sex every day and we won't catch anything. Once she starts having sex with someone else, now we can both get it. Where did it come from?

It's as though a lot of the STDs simply come from disobedience to God's sex laws; while others have a more obvious root. Seriously, if you have 10 people who don't have an STD, nobody in that group will get one as long as each of them has just 1 partner.

Once they start switching partners and getting multiple partners, that's when the STD's flare up…and you can get crabs! Isn't that crazy?

I also told you some STD's have a definite root and no matter how you try and distract society from its' root cause, you won't be able to. You won't be able to because the truth will always come to the light and facts are facts.

Do you remember AIDS and HIV? Well, I heard it started in an African country because apparently, some guy was fucking a monkey and either the monkey somehow had AIDS already or he gave the guy some type of disease that humans weren't used to. That's one theory.

I also heard AIDS and HIV came from homosexual activity that started with men having butt-sex with each other and it stayed in that brotherhood until some of them, for whatever reason, began to still get married and have wives and families…while having butt-sex with other dudes. That's another theory.

I think in all fairness, we should do some more "First 48" detective work and see what we come up with…

The monkey. I'm having a hard time with this one. 1st off, who in the fuck admitted they fucked a monkey in the ass? That's not something you would readily admit. That's one part.

Another part I'm not understanding is how did some guy fuck a monkey? Monkeys are wild animals and male monkeys don't have sex with other male monkeys. I know, I know some of you doubters out there who want to prove homosexual activity between 2 dudes is a natural thing because apparently, out of millions of monkeys and documentaries on monkeys, some unnamed monkey-watcher just happened to catch 2 male monkeys fucking each other in the butt and either caught it on tape or at least documented it and that is supposed to be all the proof needed to support homosexual activity somehow. Moving on with our wild monkey...

Monkeys are wild animals and I know humans have fucked animals before, but fucking a monkey seems too tricky to me. I watch lots of animal documentaries and even small monkeys are strong as shit and have long, sharp canine teeth!

Even if you were a professional monkey-watcher who was able to get close to monkeys and film them, a male monkey still won't let you get close enough to fuck him because that's not in their nature. That's not what monkeys do.

Am I to believe a male monkey was willing to give you a pass because you're different? You're the new guy on the block, so a male monkey decided to let you run up in his butt?

1st of all, there is a hierarchy in animal society that is similar to human society. Did you see the movie called "Friday" by Ice Cube?

In this movie, Ice Cube plays "Craig". Craig goes to visit his uncle and auntie and one day they sit around and smoke weed. While they're getting high and chit-chattin', Craig's uncle says, "Hey, nephew. You can stay with me as long as you like. Just don't touch my weed or my women."

I know that was only a movie, but there are certain household laws you have to obey to stay alive and to have a peaceful home. Who gets to fuck who is one of them.

In monkey world, the biggest male gorillas get to do all the fuckin' and they have no problem using their monkey strength to slap or body slam any other monkey who gets caught fucking or getting fucked.

With that being said, I can't imagine a dominant male allowing somebody to break protocol. I can't see him sitting back and watching while some camera guy is fucking one of the dominant male's monkeys.

Even a domesticated male monkey won't take kindly to having a dick in his butt. That's not what males in the wild do, I keep telling you. It's a fact and I wish people would stop trying to pass that one, supposed "male monkey on male monkey" sex scene off as being natural and normal.

I will say this, the chances of fucking a domestic monkey are a lot better though, than with a wild monkey. But even then, since that's not what monkeys do, you would have 2 options in my unprofessional opinion.

The 1ˢᵗ option is you would have to systematically teach your pet monkey, who is trusting you, that his butt is for sex and not for taking a shit. It would take at least 5 human years, which is probably 60 monkey years, to get where you can stick your finger in its ass and then slowly, but surely, substitute your finger for your dick.

Is it really worth it? Is it really that serious? Do you want to fuck a 60-year-old monkey in his ass that bad? And what does that say about your dick? If you can trick a monkey into thinking your dick is the same as your finger…I'm just sayin'…

So Reader, for me, the man-fucked-the-monkey theory is full of shit. What about the other theory? The theory that says 2 or more human males started having butt sex and that started to pass around a disease and it spread to women when these men got married and were on the down-low?

I think it makes sense. It actually makes perfect sense.

Your body has a specific design. Each part, each molecule, each

hair, each everything has a part. Your asshole is a part of your

body so it also has a function.

Your ass cheeks are designed to act as cushions so you can

sit down and not be uncomfortable. Since we already talked

about monkeys, I've seen them on documentaries and they have

no ass cheeks, so they look very uncomfortable sitting. It's like

their sitting with their asshole directly on the ground!

Us humans have actual ass cheeks. Somewhere near the

lower half of those cheeks is the asshole. It is "geographically"

placed where, when the time comes to take a shit, you can sit

down on your ass cheeks and comfortably take a dump.

What I'm saying is: your asshole is the shittiest part of

your body.

Your asshole is where all the waste that passes through your body goes out of.

Your asshole is designed to stay as tight as possible so that no ass-gas rudely escapes AKA a fart, at the wrong time and place.

Your asshole is where all that nasty, stinky, contaminated, bacteria-filled shit goes out your body and I'm sure little traces of that waste is right near the rim at all times.

With that being said, if I take my raw dick and continue to pump it in and out of another dude's asshole, I am guaranteed to get an infection. There is no way I can have my dick-hole open with small pieces and molecules of bacteria, waste and germs entering it…and I don't catch an STD!

I know the big thing is safe sex; especially in those settings. Question: how many of us out there know about condoms and still don't use them every, single time? If you could see me right now, you would see I have my hand raised to the fucking ceiling!

In the beginning, when the STD aspect of butt-fucking wasn't well known or documented, I can guarantee there were thousands of men getting fucked in their butts with no rubbers. I can also guarantee you that the one doing the fucking didn't wear a condom 100% of the time with his wife!

Let's do a quick recap about God's laws for sex and seafood that we've discussed so far:

1. God said don't eat seafood like shrimp because they eat shit and decaying fish and they aren't meant for us to eat. They are meant to clean the ocean and it makes sense.

2. God said don't have homosexual activity between 2 dudes because a deadly sickness will result and also, the 2 dudes aren't using their dicks, or their asses, the way He designed them. He designed the dick to be used to make babies with a woman and the asshole to get all the waste, germs, toxins and shit out of our bodies. He didn't give us this law to restrict us and not let us express ourselves

sexually and get orgasms; He did it for our health. He wants us to enjoy sex. He made us as sexual beings. He is the inventor of the orgasm. He just wants us to keep the pleasure of sex within some boundaries that allow us to have the maximum pleasure, purpose and productivity from it.

Speaking of "sex and seafood", have you noticed that the foods God told us we aren't supposed to eat *just so happen* to be the foods that are supposed to get us horny?

Yeah, I was taught eating shrimp gets your body primed for sex somehow. Ever since then, shrimp has been a goto dish for me on date-night.

Oysters is another "sex food". Cooked or smoked oysters may not be so bad, but raw oysters are downright slimy and disgusting and expensive. I swallowed them down raw thinking I was enjoying some rich-people food that would also improve my sex life. I'll tell you about it…

The 1st time I had them was in Malibu California. I had just graduated USMC bootcamp and my big brother Nick and his girlfriend at the time came and picked me up. I told them I was hungry and told them I wanted a Whopper.

I hadn't had one in months and I was craving one. They took me to Burger King and I get my Whopper.

They then took me to an apartment in, I think it was Santa Monica California near a pier. That was gonna be my spot for the night or weekend. The conversation about going out for the night came up and I was game, but I needed clothes.

They said no problem and that the Beverly Hills mall, not sure what it was called back then, was the best place to go. We get in the Benz and she asked if I wanted to drive. I said "fuck yeah" so I drove.

We left the mall and I'm not sure where I changed my clothes. I'm assuming we stopped back by "my" place in Santa Monica. From there, we took a curvy highway that I loved driving on along the coast of Malibu.

We went to a restaurant called the Gladstone, I'm pretty sure that was the name. I remember Nick and her talking about oyster shots. I never had one, but since I was fresh out of Marine Corps bootcamp, I thought I could handle anything.

The bonus for the shots was I might even get lucky that night and the oysters in my system would help my dick work properly and keep my mind focused on the sex that was gonna be happenin'.

Shit! you didn't have to tell me twice! Call the waitress and let's get it! I don't think his girlfriend did the shots. She was content to let me and my big brother catch up and do 'em.

The 1st one looked like live snot and boogers in a shot-glass! It looked disgusting, but since it was what the rich partook in and I wanted to make sure my 1st sexual experience out of bootcamp would be one to remember, I started slammin' them back-to-back with big brother.

There is a raw oyster in the glass and the glass is full of tequila. You put salt, I think, on your hand, take the whole oyster-shot in one gulp and then lick your hand to balance the strong tequila taste. I think he also put a ton of horseradish on top or made me eat a small spoonful of it which made the shots even more crazy: strong-ass tequila with strong-ass horseradish with raw-ass oyster!!

I don't remember what happened that night, but I do know I did all that shit for no reason because I was too drunk to drive home and I'm pretty sure I just passed out when I got "home".

How'd I do? Did I pretty much cover crabs, sex and STD's? Cool. Let's move on to another, fucking delicious animal God said we shouldn't eat and see why…

There are several types of animals God told us not to eat. He also told us not to eat pig. Man! I love ribs, bacon and ham! There are so many recipes and ways to enjoy the divine swine that it makes my head spin!

And yes, I had to stop eating the piggie-wiggie and the shrimp. I know it came as the result of me looking into the validity of God's laws and I know I should have just taken them at face value…but I'm just glad I got there.

What helped me realize God's law about pigs were also designed for my good? Well, for starters, I had to look at the pig's diet. They, like shrimp, are bottom-feeders. You can feed a pig anything and it will eat it.

Got a dead body you want to get rid of? Feed it to the pigs and they will eat everything except for stuff like teeth and bones.

Got some scraps from the rest of the farm? Feed it to the pigs.

Pigs, it seems, have a definite purpose and part of that purpose is waste control. That's when I had to ask myself: do I really want to eat an animal that eats shit, dead bodies and scrap food?

Here again I had to look at our typical consumer diet. We have been told the pig isn't the healthiest animal to eat, but at the same time, we have included the pig in every food and dish on the planet!

Want a nice, healthy salad? How about adding some bacon bits that come from pigs?

Want a nice, filling rib dinner? How about ordering a half-slab of pork ribs drenched in some Jack Daniels BBQ sauce?

How about a Cuban? The Cuban used to be my favorite sandwich until I realized it had ham on it and ham is another name for a pig product.

A traditional sub is a good old-fashioned ham and cheese sub. No more for me. The ham part of "ham and cheese" comes from the piggie.

My diet was taking a drastic change that I at 1st thought was for the worse until I began to fully understand 1) there is design in nature, 2) that means the Earth had a designer/creator and 3) as the designer/creator, God's laws, no matter how extreme they may seem, actually make a lot of sense!

Yeah, I couldn't eat anymore shrimp cocktail at a fancy dinner. Who gives a fuck? I'm healthier and obeying God's laws.

Yeah, I can't go to a fancy seafood restaurant and in clear conscience order some of the most expensive options on the menu. Who gives a fuck? I'm healthier and obeying God's laws.

I also got gas. Actually, we all have gas and oil or at least

access to it. We use gas every day and without it, we would all go

crazy and kill each other. We would ride around doing drive-by

shootings until we ran out of gas. It would be total chaos without

it.

Who owns all the gas and oil? Do you think Dick Cheney's

company called Halliburton owns it? What about Shell Oil or

Circle K gas? What about the nation of Saudi Arabia? If you

guessed any of those you would be right and wrong.

The truth is, they don't own shit! None of those options

actually own shit and I'll tell you why…

Who made gas? Did Shell or Circle K or the Saudis create

gas? If not, then they don't own it. They have companies that,

even though they don't take on this view, only manage gas.

Gas and oil were on this planet before humans. They are

underground in different pockets and tunnels all around the

globe. Whoever has the most money and the biggest gas-drilling operations obviously have the most and best access to large quantities of gas...but do they own it?

I'm posing this and a couple other questions to you, Reader, so you can maybe see a couple things. One thing I would like you to see is that our function on this Earth is to manage natural resources wisely.

Another thing is that no humans created natural resources, so how can any group claim to own them? That leads to what I think is going to be my final point: every natural resource we have and need every day seem to be part of Earth's design, so, we need to figure out who designed this place and learn to respect their shit!

Let's talk about gas some more. Like I already said, gas is essential to the way we live today, but it always wasn't like that.

Before the car was invented, nobody knew about gas or paid attention to gas…but it was still here in the Earth.

Once humans began to go from horses as transportation to gas-powered bikes, trucks and cars, the need to find more of this gas stuff increased. People began to no only understand its importance, they understood its importance translated to dollars and dollars translates to worldly influence, power and the amassing of personal wealth.

If you don't look at gas as being something natural that a creator or designer put here, your goal will be to control it as much as possible, use it however you want and make as money as you can off of it. Greed sets in.

For me, this hit closer to home the closer I got with God. Since I believe He is the creator/designer behind the Earth, as a sign of respect, I had to start using gas, one of His natural resources, a lot better.

This change of view is partially what helped me fully

recover from my addictions. One day I sat back and thought

about all the gas I was wasting and abusing driving around getting

high and I was ashamed of myself. I felt guilty.

Understanding and believing God owns this Earth and that

He custom-designed it and did all that planning for us to use gas

meant I had no option on how I was going to use gas.

I had to say "fuck my options" and start using my gas

wisely. I had to be aware of my gas consumption and use it only

when it was for some necessary function; particularly something

related to my purpose of creating Heaven on Earth.

Who owns the gas? Humans sure as fuck don't but we act

like we do. Common business practice says whoever owns the

land where the gas is being drilled at has rights to the gas.

Do you know where that leads me? It leads me to ask:

what humans built the land? I hope I'm not sounding too

repetitive, but you have to reach this view in order to fulfill your purpose on this planet. You *especially* have to get there if you are a business owner and more particularly a business owner in the fields of "owning" or controlling natural resources

Now, who did we say built the land? Let's use Saudi Arabia. Who built the land that Saudi sits on? I'm pretty sure they didn't and no other humans built it or the land any country is on.

Once again, you always have to follow the trail backwards as far as you can to find the motive, source or origins of a thing. Detectives are very good at this.

I routinely watch a show called "the First 48". In this show, somebody killed somebody and according to detectives, if they typically don't find a suspect in the first 48 hours after the body is discovered...they can forget about it. Their chances of finding the guilty party dramatically decreases.

One of the 1st things they do is follow the trail. Who did the victim call last? Who was the victim with? They start with questions about the victim and they progress deeper and deeper down the road to get more answers.

Once they find out who the victim was with, they question those people as though they were potential suspects and that's a good decision because trust me, on *this* show, there are some people I thought were innocent who turned out to be stone-cold killers!

When they interview potential suspects or witnesses, a lot of time the murder trail leads to money or sex. Either a potential victim has recently gotten caught cheating on his wife or the week before the victim gets killed, the victim's wife "just happened" to increase their life insurance policy from $100,000 to a payment for the beneficiaries of $500,000.

The point is, the further back you go, the clearer the truth becomes. Just like with the land the gas is on in the Saudi example, they don't own the land because they didn't create the land.

The land was there before the Saudis claimed it or won it in war. This means they really aren't the true owners of the land or the gas. Whoever actually created the land owns the land and the gas underneath it.

Once again, when you start to do your detective work and think like this, it helps you understand the beauty and design in nature and *that* hopefully leads you to start asking yourself, "Who built this planet? Why did they build it? What are their rules for operation?"

The more I began to focus on that, the less I began to focus on myself. I was becoming more and more aware that I had to, like I mentioned earlier, strive on a daily basis to stay in contact with this creator/designer to help me stay focused on my part of the plan. I just thought about something else and then we'll get back into the oil fields and stuff…

School systems and science for years has been teaching us that the universe and more specifically our planet, has no designer. We have been actively taught that there was somehow either a big explosion somewhere in a corner of the universe somehow that caused all the planets to form.

They say it took either 1 billion or 200 billion years for this process to take place. Scientists aren't really sure of the exact time frame, but they are somehow sure it happened this way.

Why am I talking about the Big Bang Theory? I'm talking about it because it is a theory that has us lost. It's a theory that wants us to believe somehow, gas, oil, water and trees somehow just happened to form on one planet out of a million planets out there.

If you are going to live with a purpose based on going as far back in time as you realistically, geographically, spiritually, naturally and historically can...you will realize there is *definitely* a creator/designer and that opens you up to acknowledging God.

And that opens us up to more questions with the main one being: since proof and facts lead to a creator/designer of this universe and more specifically planet Earth, why would our schools and the entire scientific community try and lead us away from that conclusion?

That means we gotta do some "First 48" detective work to get to the real bottom of the issue and find the perp. In this case, I am going to say the motivation for discrediting a creator/designer would be to intentionally try and use "professional" institutions like our education system and system to intentionally lead us away from the possibility that God exists and moreover, that He exists and should be getting credit for the Earth's design.

Once we acknowledge God for the Earth's design, we will then want to get to know Him on a personal level and we will begin to respect His creation and manage His resources in a respectable, responsible manner.

That leads to the creation of Heaven on Earth and that leads to humans living according to God's laws. When we actively pursue living a life according to God's laws, we turn away from evil, greedy paths of life that have Satan at the root of them.

Alright, let me slow down with the God-Satan thing. I like to not mention them so non-believers in God and the Bible are able to see the natural and most common-sense answers on their own without using the Bible.

That seems to be a common hang-up and roadblock with non-believers: how can you prove God exists by using the Bible? That line of reasoning doesn't make a whole lot of sense to me because the Bible does NOT prove God exists.

The Bible is simply a collection of reliable book, documents and manuscripts that have been recorded and passed down throughout history as examples and testimonies to God's existence. God exists whether the Bible was written or not. Let's talk some more about gas and then we'll get into the Crabs I told you I have…

What do the people who live on land they didn't make do with the profits from the gas and oil they don't own? If you want to know specifics, all you have to do is go on a channel like YouTube and type in "oil profits" or something like that.

I've done it and the things I saw were disgusting! The people who have the most control of gas and oil are taking their billions of dollars in profit to buy and personalize airplanes. Every year, they have to have a bigger and more expensive one. Right now, I think the richest one is around $1 billion dollars.

If your understanding of the Earth is that you are to control oil and gas and make huge profits and then spend the money buying billion-dollar airplanes instead of investing in something else, *anything* else, that could better improve your country or the world is crazy!

The Kings and Princes in Saudi Arabia and neighboring oil and gas rich countries are known for buying billion-dollar mansions with solid gold walls, eating utensils and toilet paper! What the fuck!?!

In case you may think I'm letting American countries off the hook because I am an American citizen, your ass is wrong! I detest and hate what large American companies like Shell and Haliburton are doing!

These companies are raking in billions of dollars of profits on foreign soil and not attempting to include the people who live in the digging territory in on the profits. America companies like

Shell Oil have no interest in supporting or helping the infrastructures of the African countries where they are digging all the natural resources from and that's disgusting.

What's equally disgusting is that back home in America, nobody in the positions to make a change give a shit. As long as America is getting as much gas as possible and our American countries are making as much money as possible...it's all good. Shell Oil is living out the great American Dream.

I'm talking about this because of the view. If a company's view is to maximize profits from the drilling, selling and controlling of natural resources, then you have greed and corruption.

You will do whatever it takes to make as much as you can and have as much control as you can over resources you don't own. You will want to take your profits and invest in your company to continue this process and be willing to spend billions of dollars on cars, houses, yachts, women and airplanes.

If a company had the view that it was simply managing those natural resources and were accountable to God for their use and the use of profits made from their sale, I think things would look differently.

Here's where I don't want to assume anything or push my view on you. I would like you to ask yourself what do you think business would look like if companies were accountable to God? Would they operate the same or would it be different? Would there still be a drive to spend billions on bullshit or towards creating Heaven on Earth? That's for you to decide on your own…

In my book, "You Don't Run Shit! a Management Story", I go into more detail about the significance of taken on a manager view over an owner view. A lot of my books share similar details and that's because I don't want you to miss anything. If you bought one book, but not a different one, you would normally

miss something and that's why I kind of cross-reference similar

topics in different books and give it to you differently.

Alright, I think that was a good, informative conversation.

What sayeth thee? All I can do is assume what your responses

and reactions are and I'm gonna assume you were enlightened,

entertained and eloquently informed.

Every book has some Private Matter Bonus Essays in it.

Either they are inserted in the Body of the book or at the end.

The essays in each book are chosen specifically for each book.

In this conversation, we talked about success and some of

Satan's hidden agendas that needed to be revealed and these

essays cover those topics. It covers those topics that people

usually like to discuss in private, hence the name Private Matter

Bonus Essays. Check 'em out:

FINDING SUCCESS the NATURAL WAY

I love to watch documentaries about animals; especially the ones about lions and tigers. For some reason I especially love to watch the life and death aspect of their lives. When I see a group of female lions getting their asses beat, I get excited. I usually get excited for one of two reasons.

The first reason is because in my YouTube video search box I typed in, "male lion attacking hyenas" and I already know what's basically going to happen and the second reason is because I have probably already watched the video a hundred times already and I already know *exactly* what's going to happen.

What's going to happen is one male lion, who is twice as big as the lionesses, is going to hear the growls and cries of pain from his lionesses and he is going to storm on the scene like a runaway freight train! He's going to grab a hyena and go straight for the jugular! Whatever hyena he attacks will be breathing its'

last breathes and I love it!

I had to finally ask myself why do I like to watch lions and

tigers kill or be killed so much? I believe I have my found my

answer, as well as a fairly reasonable explanation for my

repetitive video-watching behavior, and it's simple.

SUCCESS. That's all it is. As a human, I want to be

successful. I want to be able to do exactly what the fuck I was

designed to do. I want to be able to live on this planet in a way

that is stress free. I want to wake up every, single, mutha fuckin'

day and be excited to be alive! I want success! What does that

have to do with lions and tigers? Everything.

You see, when I watch documentaries and videos about

lions and tigers, I am watching them do exactly what it is they

were designed to do. They are called carnivores because they eat

meat. How do they eat meat?

Their eyes are positioned on their heads in such a way that they can lay low in the grass and still see the prey they are stalking. They have big ass paws with big ass claws that they will use when they jump on their prey. Once the prey is secured in place by the claws digging into its' torso, the big cat sinks its' 3-inch, sharp-as-knives, canine teeth into whatever body part is the closest.

Once the prey animal has begun to panic and slow down, the lion or tiger finds its way to the victim's throat and bites down on it, suffocating the animal to death. At this point, the attack animal's victim doesn't have a prayer. It will begin to be eaten whether it's fully dead or still alive and I love that shit!

It's a typical success scene in nature and it's what we love to see and it's what we all want to experience. Lions and tigers are predators and are built to hunt and kill and when they are doing that, they are doing what they were designed to do and there is something beautiful to see both humans and nature doing

what they were designed to do.

There is a sort of beauty and awe in it. I'm sure the prey

animals don't think so, but even them, they are doing what they

were designed to do and there is a natural beauty in that as well.

You can't have carnivores without plant-eating herbivores. And if

you didn't have carnivores, the herbivores numbers would swell

and then they would all die because since they all eat the same

grass which has a limited supply, there won't be enough to feed

all of them.

Even though I like to watch the big cats, it's to the point

where some of the videos get me so emotional and mad that I

can't watch them and that's not a good thing. It drives me

absolutely crazy because I know the wildlife photographers and

safari guides are supposed to get as close to the action as possible

to 1) make as much money from safari tours as they can and 2)

provide us with endless hours of real life animal action but still...I literally hate it and cannot watch a video where a lion is getting ready to do what it does and the safari guide has its big, bright ass light shining right on the lion, giving its position away or is driving damn near right alongside the lion just so the paying tourists can feel like they have gotten their money's worth.

I'm like, "Get the fuck out of their way!" "Stop being so close to them! Give them some space and let them breathe!" "How is he supposed to make a kill when there's 20 fucking safari trucks circling the action?!?" I literally turn the tv off and start doing pushups to take some stress off. I even have to make sure I don't talk to anybody or send an email off until I've had time to decompress properly or I might say or email off the wrong shit.

It's as though it's naturally in me to despise it when anything or anyone isn't able to freely do what it is in life. This drive for success in humans can take on some crazy forms.

This drive for success is what makes us commit suicide when we don't feel successful.

This drive for success makes us rob and steal from other people just so we can get what we want and feel successful.

This drive makes us kill each other out of greed.

This drive makes us want to do whatever it takes to get money because we feel like having money means success; and at the worst-case scenario, if we are not driven by money, we know we have to have at least a base amount to be able to survive from day to day.

I know this young buck who wants to flip houses. When I asked him why he said, "That's where the money is." And this is the part where I tie God and the Bible into this Private Matter.

If you acknowledge the facts that there is definitely natural design in life and nature and that somebody designed it, the odds of you finding success in the way it was tailor-made for you personally increases dramatically.

I believe God created everything we see and don't see. Knowing this, if He is the designer, I need to contact Him and see what His plans are for my life. The Bible is a history/law book that teaches us who God is, how we can be in contact with Him and provides plenty of examples of real-life people who were able to find their individual access by tapping into God.

I found it and I love sharing with people how it works as I go through the process. I know there aren't many examples in the upper levels of society where we see people giving God glory for their personal or financial success, but don't let that stop you. If you aren't seeing examples of humans doing what they were designed by God to do, face your life-camera to a different direction and look at nature.

In nature you will find a gazillion examples of success the way God designed it. You will see birds flying and it will give you an inner peace. It will give you a peace because even though watching a bird fly is a simple thing. Maybe you will start to see the beauty in it.

Watch a spider catch something in its web. Spiders have webs that, if they were in the human world, would be 50 times more powerful than any human-made material. Spiders naturally design different types of webs and they come with different types of venom.

Animals have God-designed weapons and skills. Each set of weapons and/or skills is designed to help each type of animal find success. After reading this Private Matter topic, I really hope you take the time to watch an animal documentary, I personally and highly recommend Big Cat videos, and look at how they are simply doing what they were designed to do.

Watching these videos might inspire you. If you're not a big animal-documentary-watcher, just watch your dog doing what it naturally likes to do and see how happy it is doing shit like licking its ass and balls or excitedly chasing its tail for 30 minutes. Watch how a baby naturally get excited just seeing you smile at it. Watch how a cat loves to irritate you by rubbing itself against your face while you sleep…knowing you are allergic to its ass. I'm a dog person but I have to admit cats are super smart…and sneaky.

It might help you properly channel that inner-drive you have for success. It might help you want to see what God, the greatest designer ever, has designed and planned for your life. Finding your personalized plan based on your design and skill will naturally lower your stress level.

You won't know until you take a look at your life from a God-design viewpoint. Your view matters, finding your God-designed purpose in life matters and you matter.

TOILET PAPER & TELEPHONES

What do you think when you read the title of this essay? At 1st glance you may think it's about talkin' shit, maybe. I mean, you got toilet paper for after you, you know what...and then you have a telephone to talk...

If you thought I would just be talkin' shit, you are wrong. I am thankful for toilet paper and telephones. That got me to thinking: all of the materials to make toilet paper and telephones was here on Earth way before they were produced. Sound boring? Take another look...

We all know there is a lot of design, law and order in nature. Somebody did a whole lot of planning in making this planet and this universe. We all know humans did not make this planet, so that means there is a 100% probability that someone out there is operating on a thought level way above our pay grade.

Toilet paper is made from paper and paper is made from trees and trees need water, dirt and sunlight to grow. If you take away any one of these elements, there is no toilet paper. Whoever designed this planet did some good-ass planning: the designer knew we humans would eventually want to wipe our asses with something softer than maple leaves or whatever they used before Charmin came around.

That's planning; especially considering how some scientist like to say the Earth was made billions of years ago. That means all the ingredients for toilet paper were put on Earth billions of years ago to be available for us to use in our lifetime.

The same can be said for the materials to make telephones, cars, bombs, windows, computers, dog food, baseball bats, pretty much everything and anything on this planet had all the materials to produce it on the Earth millions of years before any of those things were thought of. Do you now see where I'm going with this?

I believe God is the designer of the universe. With that belief, I am publicly saying He is an awesome planner and designer. He made sure everything humans would need was on this planet thousands, or millions of years ago when He made it.

Once I came to that realization, I began to trust and follow every, single plan He had and has for my life. There is no way I can make a plan today that would be fulfilled thousands of years from now. I don't have that ability. No human does.

I think it's time for us humans to humble ourselves and admit 1) there is a higher, more intelligent life form out there and 2) that life form needs to start getting the respect and honor He deserves.

I'm sticking with that life form being God. So, as a mere mortal, I had to stop stealing from Him. I had to stop robbing Him of the respect and honor that is owed to a being who operates on the level God does.

For me, that started with thanking Him for toilet paper and

telephones.

SALT and LIGHT

Salt and light are two of the most powerful and essential things on the planet. One has the ability to preserve things and the other has the power to expose things from fear to corruptions. Jesus said people who put His lessons into action should be the salt of the Earth and the light to the World. He wants His style of church to be a group of people with power and influence.

Jesus said the "Salt People" will be in charge of anything that deals with preserving the natural resources on Earth. Natural resources are not just steel, copper, plastic and water. It also includes human, animal and plant life. That means Salt People will need to do whatever they need to in order to hold any and all top positions that preserve the natural resources on Earth.

God instructed us to "maintain the Earth." This task ranges from recycling to protecting endangered wild life. It's not limited to those two tasks. They are just examples. The point is,

God needs people who want to be the Salt to maintain and

protect the Earth.

People who are destined to be the Light People have an

equally important role. They will be tasked with exposing

corruption in the world's systems. In general, light exposes things

and acts as a guide. Whenever someone is in a dark place

mentally, they need some type of light. Whenever a world system

like finance and the media, are operating and getting wealthy

based on corruption and things done in the dark, light needs to be

shown on it to expose it.

Light People have the task of holding top positions of

power in the world systems of finance, business, media,

government, religion and education to keep corruption out. At

the same time, Light People will need to be able to guide people

who are in dark places mentally. Maybe by sharing their

testimonies of how God brought them through dark times or

maybe by becoming psychologists and therapists.

Your walk in life as a Salt Person or a Light Person will be

ordained by God. What that process looks like will be different

for each person. Maybe you will be both...

Just know that Jesus said there will be a lot of people out

there who claim to want to follow Him...but the people who

actually walk the walk and talk the talk will be few...

Be a part of the few, the proud. And yes, the Marines got

that shit from Jesus.

HOMOSEXUAL ACTIVITY

I am against homosexual activity. Not because I don't like it. Not because I think it's weird. Not because I don't understand it…I am against homosexual activity because it goes against God's laws.

To be clear and fair, homosexual activity is only one of God's laws regarding sex that I am against. This may sound hypocritical, and people who are involved in homosexual activity or people who are against God, love to say that, but yes, I used to break all kinds of God's laws on sex.

God said we aren't supposed to cheat on our husbands or wives…I slept with a couple of married women in my day. That was wrong only because it went against God's laws and I had to stop. Did I want to stop? Not really, but I had no choice: it was either follow God's laws or my own laws.

God said we aren't supposed to lust. That means we aren't supposed to allow ourselves to see someone and view them as a piece of meat. I used to deal with that when I had a major porn addiction.

I would get high and watch porn for hours until my eyeballs dried up. I loved it. The rush of the endorphin releasing drug with the rush of the porn-visual had me hooked for years. I had to stop doing it. Did I want to stop? Not really, but I had no choice: it was either follow God's laws or my own laws.

People, particularly in the church, who love to point out the wrongs of homosexual activity, tend to forget about God's other laws surrounding sex. They like to point out homosexual activity while they themselves are lusting at strip clubs, hooked on porn or phone sex, cheating on their husband or wife or having sex with a very, very close family member.

This topic has been beaten up a lot and blown out of proportion. At this stage in the game, I understand 99% of humans are not involved in homosexual activity and 99% of humans don't understand homosexual activity and 99% of humans are scared to speak up and state their view because of media, personal, professional and social backlash.

I am not concerned with any of that, so I can speak freely. I follow God's laws as best as I can and I know He designed this place and that He runs shit, to if anybody has a problem with me stating my views…oh well. Get over it because I'm not stating my views, I'm stating God's views.

Anything I've done in the past that went against God's laws is something I have both an obligation to stop doing, openly confess what it is I was doing AND help people who are interested in following God's laws to stop as well. While we're on the homosexual subject, let's also be clear:

1.   there is no such thing as homophobia or homophobic. People aren't scared of people who are involved in homosexual activity. That's a very effective term that people involved in homosexual activity have used to get their "opponents" to shut the fuck up, back down and let homosexual activity become a normal thing in society.

2.   I don't call people involved in homosexual "homosexuals, gay, questioning, queer, bi-sexual, lesbian, stud, dike, fish, top or bottom" or whatever other labels are out there. I refuse to characterize someone by their sexual choices and preferences. If you like homosexual activity, you are simply a man or woman who likes homosexual activity.

3.   I am not changing my basic understanding of the English language and start calling people "him/her/she/he." That's about the stupidest, dumbest thing I could ever do. It's not that I don't respect everyone's freedom of choice…it's simply because I know how to speak English and I know that "he" is a pronoun that describes a single, individual

male. There is enough changing of the English language with words like "bad", "shit" and "lit" meaning a thousand different things. I sure as fuck am not about to start calling "him" a "her" and "she" a "he" or "me" a "him/her/he/she."

4.   Any State or country can legalize homosexual marriage, and any human who follow God's laws can not give a shit. I guess if a State says humans can marry animals that I, as a business owner, would have to start allowing spousal support for a German Shepherd's husband or wife that is an employee of mine? Get the fuck out of here. Won't happen. I operate along God's laws and am under His government's protection, guidance and care, so make whatever laws you want: if they go directly against God's laws, I will never follow them and you will never force me to.

In the end, do whatever *you* want. Suck on whoever *you* want. Fuck whoever *you* want. Marry whoever *you* want. Use fake dicks when *you* have fake sex if *you* want. Buy a fake vagina and have fake titties if *you* want...do whatever *you* want if *you* want to follow *your* own rules. When you want to wake up like I had to do and start following God's nice and easy rules for sex...let me know. I had to learn the hard way, but I might be able to help you switch over...if that's what *you* want.

Personal Development Notes